What's Happening to My Body?

A guide about Puberty and Menstruation for Girls

Joseph Nations

This guide is intended for educational and informational purposes only. The information contained herein is not intended to serve as a substitute for professional medical advice or to replace the guidance of a qualified healthcare professional. Always seek the advice of a healthcare professional with any questions you may have regarding your health or a medical condition.

Dedication

This guide is dedicated to all girls who are going through the physical and emotional changes of puberty. It's a challenging time, but also an exciting one, as you become more aware of your body and its abilities. May this guide serve as a trusted guide and companion as you navigate this period of transition, providing you with the information and support you need to feel confident, healthy, and empowered. To all the parents, caregivers, and educators who are helping young people through this important time, thank you for your support and dedication. This guide is also for you, as a tool to help facilitate important conversations and support the young people in your lives. Here's to a healthy, happy, and informed journey through puberty and beyond.

TABLE OF CONTENTS

DEDICATION

INTRODUCTION

WHAT IS PUBERTY? - A BASIC INTRODUCTION TO PUBERTY AND THE CHANGES IT BRINGS TO THE BODY.

1

MY CHANGING BODY - A CHAPTER THAT COVERS THE DIFFERENT PHYSICAL CHANGES GIRLS CAN EXPECT TO EXPERIENCE DURING PUBERTY, SUCH AS BREAST DEVELOPMENT AND BODY HAIR GROWTH.

2

UNDERSTANDING MENSTRUATION - A CLEAR AND STRAIGHTFORWARD EXPLANATION OF WHAT MENSTRUATION IS, HOW IT HAPPENS, AND WHAT TO EXPECT.

3

MANAGING YOUR PERIOD - A PRACTICAL GUIDE TO MANAGING PERIODS, INCLUDING INFORMATION ON MENSTRUAL PRODUCTS, MENSTRUAL HYGIENE, AND COPING WITH PERIOD CRAMPS.

<u>4</u>

EMOTIONAL CHANGES - A CHAPTER THAT ACKNOWLEDGES THE EMOTIONAL CHANGES THAT CAN COME WITH PUBERTY AND PROVIDES GUIDANCE ON HOW TO MANAGE THEM.

<u>5</u>

HEALTHY HABITS - A SECTION ON DEVELOPING HEALTHY HABITS THAT WILL SUPPORT OVERALL WELL-BEING, INCLUDING EXERCISE, NUTRITION, AND SELF-CARE.

<u>6</u>

TALKING ABOUT PUBERTY AND MENSTRUATION - A DISCUSSION OF THE IMPORTANCE OF COMMUNICATION AROUND THESE TOPICS WITH TRUSTED FRIENDS, FAMILY, AND HEALTHCARE PROVIDERS.

FREQUENTLY ASKED QUESTIONS - A LIST OF COMMON QUESTIONS THAT GIRLS MAY HAVE ABOUT PUBERTY AND MENSTRUATION, WITH CLEAR AND SIMPLE ANSWERS.

<u>CONCLUSION</u>

Introduction

What is Puberty? - A basic introduction to puberty and the changes it brings to the body.

Puberty is a natural process that happens to every girl as she grows up. It's a time when the body starts to change and develop from a child's body into a young adult's body. Puberty typically begins between the ages of 8 and 13, but it can start earlier or later for some girls.

During puberty, a girl's body goes through many changes. These changes happen because the body is producing hormones that cause physical and emotional changes. Some of the changes that girls may experience during puberty include:

Breast development: A girl's breasts may start to grow and become more rounded.

Body hair growth: Hair may start to grow under the arms, on the legs, and around the pubic area.

Skin changes: The skin may become oilier and more prone to breakouts.

Growth spurts: A girl may grow taller and gain weight as her body prepares for adulthood.

Menstruation: A girl's body will start to prepare for menstruation, which is when the body sheds the lining of the uterus each month.

These changes can be exciting, confusing, and even a little scary for girls. It's important to remember that every girl goes through these changes at her own pace, and there is no "right" or "wrong" way for puberty to happen.

During puberty, girls need to take care of their bodies by eating a healthy diet, staying active, and getting enough sleep. Girls should also practice good hygiene by showering regularly and taking care of their skin and hair.

Puberty can be a challenging time, but it's also a time of growth and discovery. With the right support and information, girls can navigate this time with confidence and grace.

1

My Changing Body - A chapter that covers the different physical changes girls can expect to experience during puberty, such as breast development and body hair growth.

As girls go through puberty, their bodies will start to change in many ways. These changes are a normal and natural part of growing up, and every girl will experience them at her own pace.

One of the most noticeable changes that girls will experience during puberty is breast development. As a girl's body starts to produce hormones, her breasts will start to grow and become more rounded. This can happen gradually or quickly, and every girl's experience will be different.

Another physical change that girls will experience during puberty is body hair growth. Hair may start to grow under the arms, on the legs, and around the pubic area. This is a normal part of growing up, but it can be uncomfortable or embarrassing for some girls. There are many ways to manage body hair, such as shaving or using hair removal products, but it's important to remember that there is no "right" or "wrong" way to deal with it.

Girls may also experience changes in their skin during puberty. The skin may become oilier and more prone to breakouts, which can be frustrating or embarrassing. Taking care of the skin by washing it regularly and using acne treatments can help to manage these changes.

As a girl's body goes through puberty, she may also experience growth spurts. She may grow taller and gain weight as her body prepares for adulthood. This can be a difficult time for some girls, as they may feel self-conscious or uncomfortable in their changing bodies. It's important to remember that everyone goes through growth spurts at their own pace, and it's a normal part of growing up.

Overall, puberty can be a challenging time for girls as their bodies go through many changes. It's important to remember that these changes are a natural part of growing up, and every girl will experience them in her way. With the right support and information, girls can navigate these changes with confidence and grace.

2

Understanding Menstruation - A clear and straightforward explanation of what menstruation is, how it happens, and what to expect.

Menstruation is a natural process that happens to girls and women as their bodies prepare for pregnancy. It happens when the body sheds the lining of the uterus each month, and it's a sign that the body is working properly.

The menstrual cycle is controlled by hormones that are produced by the body. These hormones cause the ovaries to release an egg each month, and they also cause the uterus to prepare for pregnancy. If the egg is not fertilized by sperm, the uterus sheds its lining, and this is what causes menstruation.

Menstruation typically lasts for 3-7 days, but it can be shorter or longer for some girls. During this time, girls will experience bleeding from the vagina. It's important to remember that this bleeding is a normal part of the menstrual cycle, and it's nothing to be ashamed or embarrassed about.

Girls may also experience other symptoms during their menstrual cycle, such as cramps, bloating, and mood changes. These symptoms are caused by the hormonal changes that happen in the body, and they can be uncomfortable or frustrating. There are many ways to manage these symptoms, such as taking pain relievers, using heating pads, and practicing self-care.

It's important for girls to have access to menstrual products, such as pads or tampons, during their menstrual cycle. These products can help to manage to bleed and keep girls feeling clean and comfortable. Girls should also practice good hygiene during their menstrual cycle, such as changing their pads or tampon regularly and washing their hands before and after handling menstrual products.

Overall, menstruation is a normal and natural part of the female reproductive cycle. It's important for girls to understand what menstruation is, how it happens, and what to expect during their menstrual cycle. With the right information and support, girls can navigate this time with confidence and grace.

3

Managing Your Period - A practical guide to managing periods, including information on menstrual products, menstrual hygiene, and coping with period cramps.

Managing your period can be a little intimidating at first, but with the right information and products, it can be a lot easier than you might think. Here are some practical tips to help you manage your period:

Menstrual Products: There are many menstrual products available, such as pads, tampons, and menstrual cups. You may need to try a few to find what works best for you. Make sure to change your pad or tampon regularly to avoid leaks and maintain good hygiene.

Menstrual Hygiene: It's important to practice good hygiene during your period. This includes washing your hands before and after handling menstrual products, changing your pad or tampon regularly, and taking a shower or bath daily.

Coping with Cramps: Many girls experience cramps during their period, but there are things you can do to ease the discomfort. Try using a heating pad or taking a warm bath, and talk to your doctor if your cramps are severe.

Dealing with Emotions: Hormonal changes during your period can sometimes make you feel emotional. It's important to take care of yourself during this time by getting enough sleep, eating healthy foods, and doing things that make you happy.

Being Prepared: It's a good idea to keep a few menstrual products with you at all times, such as in your backpack or purse. You never know when your period might start, so it's better to be prepared.

Remember, managing your period is a normal and natural part of being a girl or woman. It's important to take care of yourself during this time, and to reach out to a trusted adult or medical professional if you have any concerns or questions. With the right information and support, you can manage your period with confidence and ease.

4

Emotional Changes - A chapter that acknowledges the emotional changes that can come with puberty and provides guidance on how to manage them.

As your body goes through physical changes during puberty, you may also experience emotional changes. These changes can be challenging, but they are completely normal and temporary.

Some common emotional changes that girls experience during puberty include mood swings, irritability, anxiety, and sadness. You may also feel more self-conscious or experience low self-esteem. These emotions can be overwhelming at times, but there are things you can do to manage them:

Recognize and Acknowledge Your Feelings: It's important to recognize and acknowledge your feelings during puberty. Try to identify what you are feeling and why. This can help you better understand your emotions and how to manage them.

Talk to Someone: Talking to a trusted friend, family member, or medical professional can help you feel supported and understood. They may also be able to provide guidance on how to manage your emotions.

Take Care of Yourself: Taking care of yourself is important for both your physical and emotional health. Get enough sleep, eat healthy foods, exercise regularly, and do things that make you happy.

Practice Mindfulness: Mindfulness is a practice that can help you focus on the present moment and manage your emotions. Try deep breathing exercises, meditation, or yoga to help you feel more grounded.

Seek Help if Needed: If you are experiencing severe emotional changes or are having trouble managing your emotions, it's important to seek help from a medical professional. They can provide guidance and support to help you manage your emotions during this time.

Remember, emotional changes during puberty are normal and temporary. It's important to take care of yourself and reach out for support if needed. With the right information and support, you can manage your emotions and feel confident and happy during this time of change.

5

Healthy Habits - A section on developing healthy habits that will support overall well-being, including exercise, nutrition, and self-care.

Developing healthy habits is important for overall well-being, especially during puberty when your body is going through many changes. Here are some healthy habits you can develop to support your physical and emotional health:

Exercise: Regular exercise is important for maintaining physical health and managing stress. Find a physical activity you enjoy, such as dancing, walking, or playing sports, and aim to do it regularly. Exercise can also help boost your mood and confidence.

Nutrition: Eating a healthy and balanced diet is important for overall health. Make sure to eat a variety of foods from each food group, including fruits and vegetables, whole grains, lean protein, and healthy fats. Avoid skipping meals and try to limit sugary and processed foods.

Hydration: Drinking enough water is important for maintaining physical and mental health. Aim to drink at least 8 glasses of water a day, and avoid sugary drinks or too much caffeine.

Sleep: Getting enough sleep is important for physical and emotional health. Aim for at least 8 hours of sleep per night, and establish a regular sleep schedule to help regulate your body's natural rhythms.

Self-Care: Taking care of yourself is important for both physical and emotional health. This can include things like taking a relaxing bath, practicing mindfulness or doing something you enjoy. Self-care can help reduce stress and improve overall well-being.

Remember, developing healthy habits takes time and effort. Start by making small changes to your lifestyle, such as going for a walk each day or adding more fruits and vegetables to your meals. Over time, these habits will become second nature and can help support your overall health and well-being.

6

Talking About Puberty and Menstruation - A discussion of the importance of communication around these topics with trusted friends, family, and healthcare providers.

Talking about puberty and menstruation can be uncomfortable or embarrassing, but it's important to have open and honest communication with trusted friends, family, and healthcare providers. Here's why:

Education: Having conversations about puberty and menstruation can help you better understand the changes happening in your body. You may also learn new information that can help you manage these changes.

Support: Having trusted people to talk to about puberty and menstruation can provide emotional support and help you feel less alone during this time. They can also provide guidance and advice on how to manage physical and emotional changes.

Preparation: By talking about menstruation before it happens, you can be better prepared for when it does. You can learn about different menstrual products, how to manage period pain, and how to maintain good menstrual hygiene.

Health: Healthcare providers can provide important information about menstrual health, including how to identify abnormal periods, signs of infection, and when to seek medical attention.

Normalize: Talking about puberty and menstruation can help normalize these topics and reduce shame or embarrassment. This can help create a more open and accepting environment for all individuals.

Remember, it's normal to feel uncomfortable or embarrassed when talking about puberty and menstruation. But having open and honest communication with trusted individuals can help you better understand, manage, and normalize these changes. Don't be afraid to ask questions, seek support, or talk to a healthcare provider if you have concerns or questions.

Frequently Asked Questions - A list of common questions that girls may have about puberty and menstruation, with clear and simple answers.

Q: What is puberty? A: Puberty is a time when your body goes through many changes as you transition from childhood to adulthood. These changes can include breast development, growth of body hair, and the start of menstruation.

Q: What is menstruation? A: Menstruation is a natural process in which the lining of the uterus sheds and leaves the body through the vagina. It typically occurs once a month and is a sign that a person's reproductive system is functioning.

Q: When will I start my period? A: The age at which girls start their periods can vary, but it typically happens between the ages of 8 and 15. It's important to remember that everyone's body is different and there's no "right" age to start.

Q: How long does a period last? A: A period typically lasts between 3 to 7 days, but can vary for each person.

Q: What is PMS? A: PMS stands for premenstrual syndrome and is a group of physical and emotional symptoms that some people experience before their period. These symptoms can include cramps, mood changes, and fatigue.

Q: What menstrual products can I use? A: There are a variety of menstrual products available, including pads, tampons, menstrual cups, and period underwear. It's important to choose a product that works best for your needs and preferences.

Q: How do I manage period pain? A: There are a variety of ways to manage period pain, including taking over-the-counter pain medication, using heat therapy, and practicing relaxation techniques like deep breathing or yoga.

Q: Can I get pregnant during my period? A: It is possible to get pregnant during your period, though it is less likely. It's important to use contraception if you are sexually active and want to avoid pregnancy.

Remember, it's normal to have questions and concerns about puberty and menstruation. Don't be afraid to ask for help or seek information from trusted sources, such as healthcare providers, family members, or reliable educational resources.

Conclusion

In conclusion, "What's Happening to My Body? A guide about Puberty and Menstruation for Girls" is a valuable resource for girls who are experiencing the physical and emotional changes that come with puberty. The guide provides clear and straightforward information about what to expect during this time and how to manage the changes that are happening in the body. From understanding what puberty is and how it affects the body, to managing periods and developing healthy habits, this guide covers a range of topics that are important for girls to know as they navigate this transitional period. By providing practical advice and addressing common concerns, "What's Happening to My Body?" helps girls feel more informed and confident about their bodies and overall well-being. This guide is a must-read for any girl who is going through puberty, and it is a valuable resource for parents, caregivers, and educators who want to support young people during this important stage of development.